Your Free Gift

I want to say thank you for buying my book so I put together a free gift for you!

This gift is a perfect compliment to the book and will allow you to understand the different types of Natural Herbs! You don't want to miss out on this.

Just Visit The Link Below And Download It Totally Free!

www.lucrativelifepublishing.com//free-gift-natures-antibiotics/

I hope you enjoy this awesome treat.

Thank You For Supporting My Work.

Sydney Summers

Table of Contents

Introduction: The Troubled History of Synthetic Antibiotics

It may surprise you to know that even the ancient Egyptians and Greeks had methods for using certain kinds of mold to treat infections. One hundred years ago, infections were treated with herbal folklore remedies; only recently has mankind learned how to manipulate naturally occurring antibiotics for his benefit. Louis Pasteur famously remarked that if only man could "intervene in the antagonism observed between some bacteria", we could craft our own targeted defence against certain illnesses.

In 1942, the first heavyweight antibiotic, penicillin, was developed, and its creation was so revolutionary it won its creators a Nobel prize and place in history. The power of antibiotics to hone in on and destroy harmful elements while leaving the human body unharmed was an exciting concept.

The Bigger Picture

Unfortunately, it would seem that our understanding of how to destroy certain harmful bacteria outpaced our knowledge of the intricacies of the bacteria in the gut. It is alarmingly common for those taking antibiotics to experience a disruption in intestinal flora, which scientists are only today discovering plays a bigger role in our health than previously thought.

Diarrhea, constipation, Candida infection (thrush) and harmful bacteria overgrowth are all possible when taking antibiotics. Because the human body is composed of so many millions of kind of micro-organisms working in delicate balance, it's no wonder that a drug designed to terminate just one of them would incur some collateral damage.

What's worse, the damage wrought by antibiotics spreads further than our own bodies: antibiotics never really disappear.

Instead, they enter into the water table, damaging the environment and causing disruption that we are only just beginning to understand.

Antibiotic Resistance

Anyone with a rudimentary understanding of how evolution works will understand how antibiotics have the ironic effect of increasing the strength of the organisms it tries to kill. Bacteria live quickly and can go through thousands of generations in a very short time. This means small changes to the evolutionary path of that bacteria happen quickly - sometimes, even over the course of a few months.

If we routinely obliterate a particular bacteria, in the end, we will have no more of that kind of bacteria around. While this seems ideal, what it actually means is that we are only selecting for the best and strongest versions of that bacteria. Those that survive the antibiotic go on to replicate more, and then we have, basically, an updated version of that same bacteria. In essence, antibiotics speed the evolution of bacteria - in the wrong direction.

Penicillin, for example, used to be effective against many bacterial strains, but today its efficacy is not as great as it once was. Just as humans evolve mechanisms to defeat bacteria, bacteria evolve mechanisms to defeat humans.

While it's true that bacterial strains are always evolving anyway, the use of strong antibiotics adds a certain edge to the whole process. The use of antibiotics is one of the biggest factors leading to the development of antibiotic resistant tuberculosis, for example, or the deadly MRSE.

Antibiotic Misuse

To be fair, most doctors know that the unspoken rule with antibiotics is to use them as a last resort, and even then to not go overboard. In a perfect world, antibiotics would be used in only those cases where the drug directly and exclusively targets specific bacteria. But, we don't live in a perfect world.

Lack of understanding around how antibiotics work means people often take them without a proper diagnosis and prescription, or take them for illnesses that are actually not bacterial in nature. This harms the individual in the short term, and in the long term goes on to harm everyone by creating drug-resistant "superbugs". The strength of antibiotics increases to accommodate these new bugs, people continue to misuse *these*, and the antibiotics arms race ratchets up a notch.

What counts as antibiotic misuse?

- Using them preemptively to avoid getting sick
- Using the wrong dosage
- Taking them at the wrong time
- Not finishing the course
- Using antibiotics for everything

The worrying rise of drug resistant illnesses has many regulatory health bodies looking for ways to restrict their use, but for the time being, antibiotic misuse is rampant. Researchers are looking into ways to develop additional drugs that moderate the drug resistance in bacteria to other antibiotics - but if you think that throwing more drugs onto the problem sounds like a bad idea, then read on.

Chapter 1: What are Natural Antibiotics?

Plants are also susceptible to bacterial infection (it seems like bacteria will try their luck basically anywhere) but they deal with the threat a little differently. Plants have evolved over time to have an antibiotic film around their roots and sometimes leaves and bark, and this wards off bacteria.

Humans have discovered that the plant antibiotics available in many different herbs benefit them, too. The difference with herbal antibiotics is that they are naturally produced and much more complex than synthetic ones. While penicillin is just a single antibiotic, the compounds found in, say, garlic or yarrow plant are actually complex cocktails of many, many types of antibiotics.

This is important because it is much easier for bacteria to adapt to a simple antibiotic than it is to adapt to one that works synergistically and with an effect that is often greater than the sum of the parts.

At the risk of sounding a little too mystical, the plant has spent millennia evolving and developing bacterial resistance, just like our bodies have spent millennia developing the complicated terrain of inner flora. Against this quite ancient and infinitely complex background, it's no surprise that simple and heavy handed cures like those we've created in the last 50 years are actually not optimal.

There is an unfortunate perception that plant antibiotics and natural medicine in general is somehow weaker and less effective than synthetically prepared medicines, but in fact the strength of these medicinal plants lies in their gentleness.

A holistic approach

Herbal remedies have often been relegated to "alternatives" or merely supplements, but lately there has been growing interest in their viability. The turn to more natural remedies reflects a change in how mankind thinks of his health in general: just like the ancient civilizations before us, modern people are beginning to realize that *holistic* methods work best.

The approach of synthetic antibiotics is very simplistic, almost mechanical: diseased body minus disease equals healthy body. Right? Trouble is, disease is not something as simple as that, and so a true cure is seldom that simple, either. Treating the body like a machine or engine ignores its innate function as a system, a network of relationships and even, in the case of intestinal flora, and entire ecosystem.

To treat infections holistically, the entire body needs to be considered. Rather than popping a pill when disease strikes, building a strong immune system becomes a long term project. Together with remedial herbs, healthy foods are eaten and the healthy mechanisms the body *already* possesses are supported - constantly.

The benefits of natural antibiotics:

- Avoiding the threat of drug resistance
- Preservation of the body's natural inner balance and beneficial bacteria
- Gentle and relatively free of harmful side effects
- Cheaper and easier to obtain than commercial antibiotics
- Can be safely self administered, unlike synthetic drugs
- Can be used long term and as a part of your regular diet

In the rest of this book, we'll consider a few powerful and well-known herbs and examine their value as antibiotic tools against bacterial infection. Naturally, we need to consider those foods that also support a healthy good bacterial balance in the gut, so that the body's natural immunity is boosted even before infection happens.

We'll explore some simple and easy to prepare herbal remedies to keep at home and ways to banish harsh commercial antibiotics from your body and household right now.

Chapter 2: Natural Antibiotic Superstars

Kinds of Herbal Antibiotics

The world is teeming with botanicals that have high medicinal value as antibiotics, so the following list is by no means exhaustive. Nevertheless, the list that follows contains some of the most popular and readily available herbs.

Localized and non-systemic antibacterials are limited in their reach in the body and can't cross membranes. They are best used for GI disorders or externally on the skin, helping it to heal. A good example is Juniper berries, which can simply be brewed into a tea to heal digestive distress. Goldenseal is excellent for treating food poisoning. Included here are honey and usnea.

Synergistic herbs facilitate and icnrease the action of other plants or and herbal antibiotics. An excellent examples is ginger root. Brew a tea of fresh slices for colds, nausea and abd circulation. Other examples include black pepper and licorice, especially the root.

Systemic Herbs, as the name implies, treat whole systems, and are good for addressing staph infection, TB and malaria.

• Cryptolepis, sida, alchornea, bidens and artemisia are the 5 popular herbs in this category and are usually taken on a very specific program. It's best to work with a trained herbalist when using these herbs.

It is not terribly important for you to know and understand a plant's chemical make-up, category etc. for you to benefit fro its use, however its wise to pay attention, as always, to the way herbs affect you – the gold rule is to always listen to your body.

Calendula

This gorgeous orange flower gets its name from the same Latin root word for "calendar". Calendula is also known as marigold and many people have no idea that the pretty blooms in their garden are actually medicine. Calendula is primarily used externally as a poultice for stings, burns and skin disorders and contains powerful plant compounds that fight infection.

Cinnamon

Cinnamon is so delicious that people can underestimate its medicinal properties. Cinnamon is warming and incredibly balancing for the blood sugar levels. Cinnamon has excellent antibacterial properties and can be applied to the skin directly if blended with a carrier oil to moderate its strength.

Clove

Another culinary herb that has underrated medicinal value. Clove is particularly beneficial for fighting Candida overgrowth and has direct and powerful effects on certain strains of intestinal bacteria.

Garlic

Garlic contains over 120 naturally occurring antibacterial plant compounds, making it more broad spectrum than something like penicillin. Garlic can be taken in many forms, although raw is best as high temperatures start breaking down the valuable plant proteins. Garlic is excellent as it leaves your beneficial bacteria perfectly intact, and is best eaten in small regular doses. Add liberally to food and consider taking capsules of dried powder.

Echinacea

Several ancient peoples independently learned to appreciate the value in this beautiful purple plant. Colds, flus, strep throat and abnormal pap smears all respond well to echinacea's blend of plant antibiotics. Many use echinacea prophylactically; it's a great supplement to take daily during cold season.

Marshmallow root

Marshmallow contains plant tannins that are quite useful in protecting the urinary tract and is very useful for infections in this area. A great addition to blends intended to reduce pain, too.

Yarrow

This unassuming herb is actually a darling of antibiotic herbs and has many uses. A tea of yarrow is great for urinary tract infections, fighting sepsis and speeding healing.

Aloe

Aloe is often assumed to be only a topical treatment but has great benefits internally, too. Externally, a piece of fresh aloe soothes and heals burns and skin infections, and when taken internally, is effective against many bacterial strains, including herpes simplex (responsible for cold sores).

Eucalyptus

Eucalyptus oil is a potent decongestant and is very effective at clearing away mucous and calming and soothing inflamed cells - perfect for colds and flus, although should not be taken internally.

Usnea

A massively versatile localized herb that treats staph and strep strains, all breathing and sinus infections and also viral infections such as in vaginosis.

Sage

Excellent for sore throats and a great anti-inflammatory. Reduces mucous.

Licorice root

Good against strep and staph infections, TB, candida albicans, E coli, salmonella and even malaria. Licorice root stimulates the body's own immune system and is great for soothing a sore throat. Licorice root is powerful and should be used with caution in those with high blood pressure.

Chapter 3: Strengthening the Immune System Naturally

Before we move onto useful ways to combine the above herbs into preparations that you can use to help prevent and treat bacterial infection, we should look at the other side of the equation: your body's own immune system. Sicnreaseicnrease you already have a sophisticated system in place designed to deal with bacterial threats, it makes sense to get the most out of this system.

What follows are some foods and supplements that are not necessarily herbal but serve to boost and enhance the body's immunity by populating the gut with beneficial bacteria. The gut is a crowded place - if you are well populated with beneficial bacteria, it will be much more difficult for harmful bacteria to gain a foothold.

Your immunity rests in your intestinal lining

Many people don't at first understand how good digestion is connected to immunity, but your body's ability to defend against attack occurs in large part in the gut lining. Proper digestion is the first line of defense, and when it its compromised, a domino effect of infection and inflammation is set up.

"Leaky gut syndrome" occurs when the membrane lining the gut becomes too porous. This happens when harmful plant proteins (such a gluten or things like lectin and phytate in grains) eat away at the lining. The tiny holes permit undigested particles of food directly into the bloodstream, where they cause the body to respond defensively - often by creating histamine to deal with the inflammation.

Food allergies, malabsorption, bloating, constipation and diarrhea, frequent infection etc. are all symptoms of a compromised gut immune system. When the immune system is so busy fighting off infections merely from food, there is less energy to respond to true infections. The body fills with inflammation and cortisol, hormone levels are disrupted, blood sugar levels are thrown off balance and the result is an entire body that is unwell and functioning well below optimal.

Gut bacteria make up, by number, more cells and more genetic material than the cells that make up your own body. They are responsible for ensuring the smooth functioning of every enzyme and hormone involved in the complicated process of digestion. Poor immunity starts in the gut, and to heal autoimmune disorders, a propensity to frequent colds or infections, healing has to start in the gut.

How do you heal leaky gut?

Reintroducing healthy bacteria into the system is the first line in treating an inner ecology that is out of whack. What follows are some foods that encourage healthy bacterial growth in your intestines and promote the healthy function of your immune system.

Coconut oil

One of the most potent antiviral, antifungal and antibacterial treatments. Whether eaten or applied topically, it's almost as if coconut oil was designed specifically to promote healthy bacteria in the gut and kill of the unhealthy kind. Medium chain fatty acids in the oil, specifically lauric acid, break down and attack directly the cell walls of bacteria and viruses, killing them off. What's more, coconut oil soothes and heals an inflamed gut lining, stabilizes blood sugar and aids in hormone regulation.

Coconut oil is an amazing daily supplement. Eat a tablespoon each morning by itself, or else add it to cooking, in smoothies or even externally as a soothing balm. There is almost nothing coconut oil cannot do, and natural healers have used it for arthritic pain, eczema, diabetes and obesity, treating candida (internally and topically) and much more. Bacterial "die-0ff" will occur with a dedicated regime of about 3 tablespoons per day. Make sure your oil is organic, cold pressed, unhydrogenated and unrefined.

Fermented vegetables

A happy side effect of the ancient technique of preserving and pickling veggies is that fermented food is excellent at repopulating the gut. Any fermented vegetables (not store bought, but preferably homemade) contain acids, enzymes and beneficial bacteria. Sauerkraut and Korean kimchi are delicious and can be eaten often. They're low carb, low fat and bursting with vitamins and minerals anyway, so find a place for them in your diet.

Fermented dairy

In the same way, fermented dairy allows helpful bacteria to set up colonies in your gut that repel infection and ease proper digestion. Choose proper yogurt with cultures, sour milk or kefir, which you can make at home easily if you have the "grains". These grains can also be used to make water or coconut milk kefir.

Commercially available probiotics

It's also possible to simply take capsules of beneficial probiotics directly. Make sure they have a high probiotic count (above 5 million units if possible) and take regularly.

Bone broth

Finally, bone broth or stock is a vastly underrated health food that can quickly heal a tattered gut lining and promote a truly resilient and healthy immune system. Bone broth contains dozens of beneficial fatty acids, minerals and vitamins, as well as soothing collagen and compounds that "heal and seal" the intestinal lining.

Leaky gut can be cured within 3 or 4 days eating bone broth alone to give the body time to rest and rebuild its immune defense. This is also an excellent treatment for allergies, overweight and autoimmune disturbances. Think of it as a reset button for your gut.

A recipe will be included later, but bone broth can be boosted by including healing and antibiotic herbs to the mix, as well as taking some coconut oil each day to help along the healing.

Chapter 4: Healing Herbal Recipes

Once you realize how easy it is to make your own healing herbal tinctures, teas, poultices, rubs and bath soaks, you'll wonder how you ever relied on conventional treatments in the first place. A well stocked herb pantry offers a remedy for practically any health problem, and you get the peace of mind of knowing that you are not contributing to growing mutant bacterial strains or harming your own internal balance.

A word of caution though: herbal medicines are still medicines. Though their action is milder and more cumulative than conventional medicines, it is still more than possible to overdose, to take a herb that is not meant for you or to combine herbs that don't really belong together.

If you have a pre-existing medical condition, the onus is on you to ensure that the herbs you take will not interfere with your condition or any of the medication you are taking to treat it. For the most part, herbs taken during pregnancy and lactation are risky and this should only be done under the close supervision of a herbalist or naturopath that you trust.

As with anything that you put into your body, start small and then take note of how your body responds. Gradually increase the dose and be vigilant. Stop if you experience bad side effects - some people do have sensitivities to certain herbs. Don't attempt to try herbal remedies without eating healthily and living well at the same time - herbs taken on top of addictions, substance abuse or a very unhealthy diet are not going to be able to help much.

Lastly, be patient. Herbal remedies are almost never quick fixes and many remedies take around a month of daily use to start having an effect. Keep at it.

Right! Now that we've covered the fine print, let's move onto the actual recipes. Below are some healing recipes organized according to the symptoms they'll treat or else what their general function in the body is.

Recipes for Soothing Colds and Flus

Echinacea and Yarrow Tea

Simply brew a few teaspoons of dried echinacea leaves and roots as well as equal parts dried yarrow to make a tea. Drink throughout the day.

Thyme tea

Make a tea from fresh thyme or thyme oil to fight colds and flus. It isn't pleasant tasting but it is effective against infection. Can also be rubbed onto the skin with a carrier oil.

Recipes for Supporting the Immune System

Garlic soup

Most people don't need much encouragement to add more garlic to their cooking, but ramp up your intake in the winter months to give your body a boost in immune function. First, take the top fifth of a whole garlic head off with a very sharp knife, just so that each clove is exposed. Do this with three garlic heads and coat the exposed ends with olive oil. Roast until golden and soft, about an hour.

Now, gently take each clove out of its pocket with a butter knife and blend with chicken or vegetable broth, cream, salt and pepper. This will make a thick, rich but very mild soup loaded with garlicky goodness. Garnish with toasted ciabbatta bread and a good sprinkle of fresh parsley.

If you're impatient and like your garlic a bit more rustic, simple serve the garlic heads as the centre piece of a cheese board - everyone can help themselves to the freshly roasted cloves. Serve with bread, cheese and good red wine.

Basic Bone Broth

This recipe is endlessly adaptable, but is a good basic stock to work with and add your own creative touch to. You'll need:

1 chicken carcass, meat removed, or a selection of beef bones
A large stock pot
1 Onion
1 Carrot
1 Celery Stalk
3 or 4 Bay Leaves
Spices: Pepper, chilli, dried herbs, juniper berries
A few tablespoons of apple cider vinegar

To make the broth, make sure your bones are completely submerged in water. Add the vinegar (this helps leech the minerals out of the bones) and spices (remember not to add salt - yet). The vegetables and bay leaves are added (raw or previously roasted), the water brought to a boil and then simmered for 3 to 4 hours, or until the broth is lovely and golden in color.

If the broth reduces too much, add more water and lower the temperature. Don't worry about fat bubbling to the surface - this isn't pretty to look at but it shows the healing collagen and fatty acids are being released. Try to skim off the "scum", which is grey and non-fatty looking.

Strain the contents of the pot and retain the liquid. The vegetables can be thrown away or put onto a compost heap, and the very soft bits of tissue can be fed to pets provided there are absolutely no sharp bits that can hurt them. Also remember not to give pets onion.

Don't worry about it if your broth is cloudy or very thick - this is likely a good thing. Your stock can be frozen, refrigerated or used is another recipe. Broth alone with a little salt and some turmeric and ginger is an amazing (and delicious!) immune system booster and will help you fight off colds and parasites, as well as healing your gut.

Alternatively, have the occassional day where you only drink warm broth and other liquids to detox and rest your system, or make the quintessential chicken soup to treat a cold - load it up with good protein, vegetables and plenty of healing herbs.

Vitamin C Tea

This is a strong flavorful tea filled with antioxidants and beneficial plant phytates - it tastes amazing, too.

Combine crushed rosehip shells with cinnamon chips, lemongrass, fennel seeds and hibiscus in the ratio 4:2:2:2:1. Whole rosehips can be used, or you can try brewing the crushed shells, which have a greater surface area and don't need to brew for as long. Steep for up to 10 minutes and sip throughout the cold and flu season or to treat a head cold.

Recipes for Treating Bacterial Infections

To treat candida

Begin a program of coconut oil to encourage bacterial die-off. Work your way up to two or three tablespoons a day at least. Coconut oil can also be applied topically.

Curry

You might not think of this as medicine, but certain curries are bursting with antioxidants and antiviral and antibacterial plant compounds. Make a curry paste by combining ginger, garlic, tamarind, onion, chill (particularly cayenne pepper), black pepper, turmeric, cinnamon, anise, clove, cardamom, lemon juice and even a bit of coconut oil. Add tomatoes and a little cream or coconut milk to make a sauce and serve piping hot over basmati rice or alone.

Oregano oil gargle

Mix a few drops of oregano oil in water and gargle to treat a throat infection. Not for pregnant women. Can also be swallowed for a cold and flu treatment as oregano oil is a potent antiviral.

To treat drug-resistant staph infection

Use 1 teaspoon of dried Cryptolepis plant in a teapot and allow to steep for 10 minutes. One to two cups will prevent onset and up to 6 cups can be taken in acute cases of staph infection.

You can get similar results by also using dried Sida and preparing and drinking in the same way. In acute cases, up to 10 cups of Sida tea can be taken per day to fight infection. Both of these herbs are quite difficult to get hold of in the United States especially, but if you do your research you can find online suppliers and vendors – just be sure to do your homework and be careful about what you're buying.

Recipes to Treat the Respiratory System

Cough and sore throat tea

This tea will actually help fight mucous build up in the sinuses, calm a sore throat and help reduce coughs, especially wet or "chesty" coughs.

Blend equal parts of dried lemongrass, sage and lime blossom, also know as linden blossom. Brew a tea from this blend for around 5 - 8 minutes and then sip slowly for relief of a sore throat. Can also be served cold or with honey and lemon.

Honey, ginger and lemon drink

Mix a spoon of honey, a squirt of fresh lemon and a few slices of fresh ginger in a cup and add piping hot water to mix. Sip this while it's still very hot, ideally before bed. Delicious, soothing and antibacterial. Also good for sore throats and congestion.

Healing Vapor

Put a few drops of rosemary, camphor, eucalyptus and tea tree oil in a bowl of just boiled water. Close your eyes and put your head over the bowl, covering with a towel and breathing deeply. This will open up tight chests and relieve congestion and blocked noses.

To make a healing vapour bath, you could fill a small muslin bag with dried rosemary, eucalyptus or camphor leaves and let it float in a very hot bath. The steam will relieve congestion and soothe muscle aches. Avoid putting neat oils directly into the water as some of these can burn the skin.

To make a healing rub, combine a few drops of the above oils into a base of either grapeseed, olive or coconut oil and then rub onto the chest and the back, to open up congestion. Alternatively, a few drops of the oil can be put onto a handkerchief or tissue and inhaled.

Recipes to Treat the Skin

Coconut skin treatment

Coconut is a beautiful antiviral, antibacterial and antifungal medicine and can be used with great success inside and outside the body. If you're battling dry skin, eczema, psoriasis, acne or any other skin condition, coconut oil will likely help you. Try this treatment once a week or as often as you need it, adjusting to suit your needs.

You'll need:
A tablespoon of cinnamon
A cup of brown sugar
Enough melted coconut oil to make a paste

Combine the above ingredients to make a scrub. In the shower, gently use this mixture to slough away at dead or dry skin. Both of these ingredients will cleanse the skin and treat any surface infections, and the cinnamon will increase blood flow, bringing a rosy glow as you gently scrub with the sugar. Rinse, then once you're out of the shower, coat your entire body with a thin layer of pure coconut oil once again, to seal in the treatment. Don't be too generous, as a little goes a long way. You can combine aloe gel or camphor if you have it on hand.

This treatment also works wonders on sore joints or osteoarthritis. Coconut oil is one of the few substances that can penetrate the sealed joint and work at infections there that cannot be accessed by conventional antibiotics. The medium chain fatty acids do not need to enter via the bloodstream and can be absorbed quickly, lubricating and disinfecting the joint. Take some time to massage problem areas.

What many people don't know is that dandruff is often caused by tiny parasites burrowing into and irritating the surface of the scalp. Moisturizing the scalp in this case will simply not address the underlying cause.

If persistant dry scalp, itching or drynes is a problem, this treatment can help:

Make sure you are using a sulphate free and gentle shampoo. Avoid medicated kinds as these can be very harsh. Otherwise use a simple homemade shampoo or castille soap blended with lavender oil, or a solution of bicabonate of soda. In the extreme, many people find relief from gradually weening themselves off of shampoo entirely and relying only on water to cleanse, although this takes some time for the hair to adjust.

After washing, rinse the hair in a solution of around 3 tablespoons of apple cider vinegar, some brewed nettle tea (the longer it's brewed, the better) and a few drops of rosemary oil or else a strong rosemary decoction made of fresh leaves. Mix with enough water in a jug to make a rinse that can be poured over the head.

Don't rinse with water after this. The vinegar smell will dissipate as the hair dries. These ingredients will get to work toning and clearing the scalp, and rosemary adds extra shine and gloss to hair. If you like, you can precede this whole treatment with a coconut oil hair mask: generously rub the oil into the scalp and allow it to sit for an hour or so before you wash your hair.

Though most people think of acne as some sort of cosmetic problem, the skin is in fact an organ just like any other, and acne is a manifestation of that organ's stress and malfunciton. From the inside, acne can be treated by drinking nettle tea (especially if the acne is hormonal in nature - i.e. is cyclical in women or else centred repeatedly on one area of the face, commonly the chin). Zinc and omega 3 supplements help acne in all cases as does eating food high in both - oily fish in particular.

From the outside, try an antibacterial regime to make sure your skin is bacteria free, clean and soft. In the morning, cleanse with honey, an ancient and powerful antibacterial beauty aid. Mix a bead of honey with a little water to thin - the water activates small amounts of hydrogen peroxide in the honey and this is cleansing and slightly lightening for the skin.

Make sure you don't get any water into the honey jar as it will spoil. Cleanse the face and rinse with warm water. Use your usual moisturizer or a thin layer of coconut oil. At night, do oil cleansing, another excellent acne treatment that cures people of horrible pustules without having to rely on harsh synthetic chemicals.

Here's how: moisten the face. Spread a layer of olive oil onto the skin and massage for a few minutes to break down oil (oil dissolves oil). Have the tap running until the water is as hot as you can stand it, then wet a facecloth with this water and quickly lay the cloth over your face to "steam". Don't rub, just pat. Then, repeat the process again, at least 4 or 5 times. This cleans away oil on the surface of the skin without drying it. On the final round, scrub a little to get rid of residue and dry. No need for a moisturizer.

This treatment works because often, acne prone skin is both too oily and incredibly dry - drying treatments only force the body to create more sebum and the cycle continues. Keep up this regime for a month and you will notice a definite improvement. Tea tree oil can be dabbed on pimples to treat them directly.

To treat burns or rashes

Run a lukewarm bath with marigold (calendula), aloe and camphor to soothe sunburn. You can add these directly as the whole herb (put into a bag to make clean up easier) or you can brew a tea and then add that to the water. Soak a while and then smooth a mixture of coconut oil and aloe vera gel on the affected areas. Make sure to drink plenty of water.

To treat wounds

A thin layer of either honey or coconut oil spread around the edge of a cut, scrape or even bruise will seal the area off from infection and prevent dust and microorganisms from entering. Much better than a band aid!

Recipes That Use Herbal Essential Oils

The following remedies are delivered directly into the body through capsule form and so are great for oils that would be too potent to use as a tea or eaten directly. Look round online or buy size "00" capsules from a health food store that you fill yourself.

"Thieves" Antimicrobial Flu Blend

This historic blend reportedly helped a band of French thieves avoid contracting plague while they robbed its victims. Combine equal parts of clove oil, cinnamon oil, lemon oil, eucalyptus oil and rosemary oil. You could also buy a commercially available "thieves oil" blend which may contain different ratios. Mix the oils and put into capsules. Take one capsule every 3 or 4 hours when you notice the first flu symptoms and then taper off as your symptoms subside.

This blend works because the ingredients are antibacterial, antifungal, anti-infectious, antiparasitic, antiseptic, antiviral and stimulating for the immune system. The above can also be combined with a small amount of oregano oil, thyme oil or frankicnreasense oil if you have them on hand. Drink plenty of fluids and rest and you'll be good to go.

Herbal Parasite Cleanse

Many people don't think too much about parasites, but worms, microorganisms and other parasites in the body can be incredibly destructive and are more common than you think. Many herbalists make a habit of completing a yearly or half yearly cleanse to make sure that their bodies are free of harmful parasites.

Take together a capsule of clove oil, a capsule of wormwood oil and a tincture of black walnut hull. These can be found in health food stores or else complete kits can be bought online. IMPORTANT: this herbal remedy is extremely potent and you should never attempt to mix it yourself, as the results can be deadly. Speak to a trained herbalist first. Also to be completely avoided if you are pregnant or breastfeeding. Wormwood oil has been known to cause renal and liver failure so again, be *very* careful when handling these herbs.

Conclusion

Thank you again for downloading this book!

Hopefully in this short book you've been inspired to find natural and simple ways to treat colds, flus and infections. With a little care and foresight, you can find everything you need to treat viral and bacterial infections in nature, without having to resort to harsh and even harmful synthetic antibiotics.

If you are just starting out with antibiotic herbs, try some of the simple recipes outlined here and gradually work your work up to more complicated blends with the help of a professional herbalist. Nothing can beat the sense of satisfaction that comes with working *with* your body in natural and wholesome ways.

A healthy lifestyle goes a long way to supporting your body's own natural immunity, but even in the event of an infection, natural antibiotics work quickly and safely, without disrupting your body's balance or creating drug resistance in the bacteria themselves.

Finally, if you enjoyed this book, would you mind leaving me an honest review? Reviews are so important for authors like me and it would mean a huge amount to me if you took the 2 minutes to write one.

I do look forward in reading your review, thanks in advance.

Also, if you missed your Free Gift just flip to the next page to get it now!

Your Free Gift

I want to say thank you for buying my book so I put together a free gift for you!

This gift is a perfect compliment to the book and will allow you to understand the different types of Natural Herbs! You don't want to miss out on this.

Just Visit The Link Below And Download It Totally Free!

www.lucrativelifepublishing.com//free-gift-natures-antibiotics/

I hope you enjoy this awesome treat.

Thank You For Supporting My Work.

Sydney Summers

www.ingramcontent.com/pod-product-compliance
Lightning Source LLC
Chambersburg PA
CBHW060445290526
45793CB00002B/579